W9-CEA-087

30 DAYS TO A BETTER BUST

////////////////////////////////

A no-nonsense guide to making the most of what nature gave you and to feeling great about yourself

BY
REGINA LARKIN AND JULIE DAVIS

BANTAM BOOKS
TORONTO · NEW YORK · LONDON · SYDNEY

DESIGNED BY JON DEWEY
PHOTOS BY RON CONTARSY
ILLUSTRATED BY ELAINE YABROUDY

/ / / / / / / / / / / /

ACKNOWLEDGMENTS

We would like to thank Jeff Nayer, our favorite weight lifter, for his invaluable assistance. Jeff generously offered his time and experience in putting together the Terrific Twelve program of shape-up exercises used in this book and in answering our many questions about weight training for women.

/ / / / / / / / / / / /

Before starting any new exercise or diet program, it's always best to have a medical checkup. This is a must if you have any serious medical conditions or if you are taking medication. Call your doctor before you begin.

---

30 DAYS TO A BETTER BUST
A Bantam Book / October 1982

All rights reserved.
Copyright © 1982 by Cloverdale Press, Inc.

This book may not be reproduced in whole or in part, by mimeograph or any other means, without permission.
For information address: Bantam Books, Inc.

ISBN M-01488-9

Published simultaneously in the United States and Canada

Bantam Books are published by Bantam Books, Inc. Its trademark, consisting of the words "Bantam Books" and the portrayal of a rooster is Registered in U.S. Patent and Trademark Office and in other countries. Marca Registrada. Bantam Books, Inc. 666 Fifth Avenue, New York, New York 10103.

PRINTED IN THE UNITED STATES OF AMERICA

0 9 8 7 6 5 4 3 2 1

TABLE OF CONTENTS

INTRODUCTION

30 DAYS TO A BETTER BUST is a complete guide to improving the look of the breasts. It combines a program of muscle-toning exercises with beauty and fashion advice to make you look terrific.

There are no gimmicks involved. Unlike the kits advertised in magazines, unlike hypnotism techniques, or even the latest bust-building fad in which electric waves are shot under the skin, we don't pretend to increase your measurements dramatically or by magic.

Ours is an integral straightforward plan designed to raise and shape the bust. It takes effort on your part (you'll find that the results increase with your dedication), but it's fun, too. Most of all, 30 DAYS TO A BETTER BUST will help you feel good about yourself—and make you your sexiest ever!

1. BE STRONGER, BE SEXIER

Every woman is concerned about her figure, especially her breasts, often equating her self-worth with that one measurement. The problem isn't just physical, it's emotional, too. Yes, it's great to have the best figure you can, but it's even more important to feel great about the figure you do have.

Your first goal is to have a better attitude. Too many women are overly critical of themselves, believing that they don't measure up to one ideal or another, the sensuality of a sex symbol, say, or the sleekness of a fashion model. (This is true of women who are amply endowed as well as women who feel they have shortcomings!) A negative self-image is defeating, so take a positive and practical approach instead. Tell yourself that you will do everything you can to look your best and that you will be satisfied with your efforts. Determine the amount of energy, both physical and mental, that you're willing to devote to this part of your body, and decide that you're going to look fabulous. Always remember that you mustn't compare yourself to anyone else. You're an individual, you're special, and the only person you have to please is yourself.

Your second goal is physical improvement. By developing the contours of your upper torso, you can improve the appearance of your bust and, even more important, increase your strength. Too often, women don't give their arm, shoulder, and chest muscles a good workout. Toning the muscles in these areas is a must to prevent or postpone flabby upper arms and sagging breasts, frequently among the first signs of aging.

We've come a long way in getting equal status with men; now we're at the last frontier: strong enough to tote our own bags and open our own jars! There is a great natural zestful feeling that comes from experiencing our own strength, a feeling all women can have with just a little upper-body work.

We know the breasts themselves are made up largely of fatty tissue. However the muscles surrounding the breasts serve as a support and can be developed to make the breasts appear higher and firmer, no matter what their size. The way to tone and build these muscles is with exercise, specifically a series of exercises using weights.

Don't worry about becoming a female Arnold Schwarzenegger. It's not possible for you to become muscle-bound or unfemininely *pumped up*. To develop a body builder's massive proportions, the body needs testosterone, a hormone predominant in men. Not even female body builders who spend hours at a stretch pumping iron can achieve such dramatic results.

The 30 DAYS TO A BETTER BUST plan takes less than 30 minutes three times a week. You work out every other day (Sundays are always free). There's no chance of your becoming overdeveloped in these few sessions, but the workouts will

- improve your figure
- tone your muscles
- increase your strength . . . in a beautiful way

Along with a positive attitude and physical activity, your personal style will help you have the figure you've always wanted. The clothes you wear can improve the results of the exercise program. We're not talking about padded bras, either, but a carefully chosen wardrobe to flatter your natural assets.

How you care for yourself counts too. Most women stop their beauty care at the neck. Your skin should feel satiny smooth from your head to your toes. Taking a few extra minutes to pamper yourself can make all the difference in the way you feel about yourself and, therefore, in the way others perceive you.

★For some women, nothing short of cosmetic surgery will do. Fooling with Mother Nature is a drastic step to take. If you've ever wondered about breast surgery, your questions will be answered in a special chapter devoted to this subject.

2. PERFECT PECTORALS...AND MORE

///

To improve the appearance of your bust, you need to work not only the pectoral muscles, but also the serratus muscles underneath the breasts, the deltoid muscles of the shoulders, the latissimus dorsi of the back, and the triceps and biceps of the upper arms. The Terrific Twelve is a series of exercises designed to get all these muscles working. Together, these muscle groups create a more beautiful definition of the contours of your upper torso. More than just a better bust, you'll also develop graceful shoulders, shapely upper arms, and a slender back. Be sure to do all 12 exercises faithfully.

Each of the 12 exercises is a weight workout. All call for pressing and lifting dumbbells. When done correctly, weight-training exercises produce faster and more noticeable results than exercises done without them, because the muscles have to work harder. The basic weight of each of the dumbbells you'll be using is five pounds, well within the range of most women. But for your own well-being, do get your doctor's approval before starting this or any other exercise program.

HOW TO SELECT FREE WEIGHTS

Free weights are weights used independently of weight-lifting machines such as the Nautilus and Universal models. They include weight cuffs that strap onto the ankles and wrists, dumbbells used in either hand, and barbells lifted with both hands.

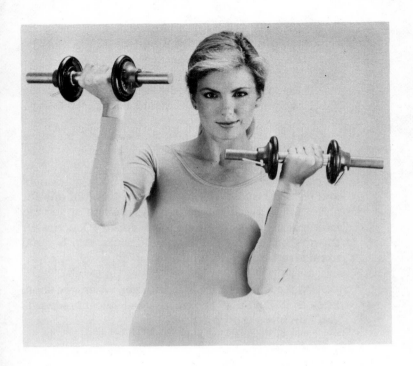

The Terrific Twelve exercises call for two dumb-bells, which can be purchased at any sporting goods store. Because the weight requirement for the individual exercises varies slightly, it is best to have dumbbells that can be adjusted. Here's what you need:

* two 5-lb. dumbbell bars.

* sleeves and collars to hold weights in place.

* four 1¼-lb.-weight plates or discs to bring the weight of each dumbbell to 7½ lbs. (The sleeve and collar together weigh 1¼ lbs.)

* four 2½-lb.-weight plates or discs to bring the weight of each dumbbell to 10 lbs.

As your strength increases, you can add on more weight. But progress slowly and carefully.

The only other equipment you'll need is a bench. You should be able to buy a relatively small one for about $25. However, you can use a piano or sewing bench instead. An ironing board placed 10 inches off the ground (use two fat telephone books at either end to raise it) also works well.

Make a list and bring it with you when you shop. Stick to it. Don't let an overzealous salesperson talk you into more than you need.

HOW TO GET STARTED

* Exercise *every other day*, three times a week. Weight exercises *break down* the muscle tissue. (This might sound harsh, but it isn't.) Your body needs time to rebuild this tissue.

* On alternate days, practice an aerobic sport to round out your physical training. See page 42 for the best choices.

* Wear a good sports bra and support sneakers when working out. Caring for your body includes protecting it, and these two sportswear items do that job well.

* Follow the directions and carefully note placement of the hands, the feet, and the weights in each photograph. Do your exercises in front of a mirror to make sure you maintain the right form.

* Note the muscle group each exercise reaches. If you feel the workout in the right place, you're doing the exercise correctly. If you don't, check your form.

* Control your breathing. When to inhale and when to exhale are noted in each exercise. For best results, breathe in through your nose and blow out through your mouth. By concentrating on your breathing, you'll put more effort into each exercise.

* The heavier the weight, the harder you'll have to work to lift it—and the sooner you'll reach your goals.

* Do each repetition slowly. Let your body return to its full starting position before going on to the next rep. Don't watch the clock, watch your body. Be thorough and careful and you will see great results in just 30 days!

THE WARM-UP

Warming up before any type of exercise prevents sprains and enables you to work at your peak. Take the time to warm up before your weight work, with the following exercises:

1. Shoulder shrugs.

Raise your shoulders until they touch your ears (almost!). Hold for one second, then release. Reps: three sets of five.

2. Shoulder rotations.

Bring your shoulders up to your ears, then pull them back, then down, then around to their natural position.

Reps: five rotations clockwise, five rotations counterclockwise.

3. Arm rotations.

Stand with your arms at your sides and bring them up to shoulder level. In a clockwise direction, make ten circles with your arms. Start with a small circle and work up to the largest one you can make. Reverse direction, making smaller and smaller circles until you are back at the starting position.

Reps: repeat the entire exercise three times.

4. Jumping jacks.

Do 25 of these to pump the blood to your muscles.

THE TERRIFIC TWELVE

Do each exercise that follows. Aim for the full number of repetitions within the sets, but, again, always maintain the proper form, even if this means completing only one set at first. You'll improve with practice.

Try not to stop for more than a minute between sets or between exercises. Your workout should be done in one continuous period.

Remember that you will be working out only three times a week. Make these times count!

ONE
DUMBBELL BENCH PRESS///////////

for the pectorals

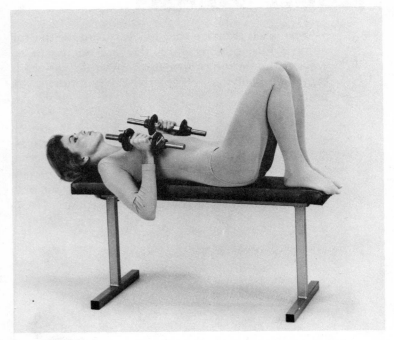

  1. Sit at the very edge of your bench, feet together, and flat on the floor. If your feet don't comfortably reach the floor, bend your knees and place feet flat on the bench. Hold a dumbbell upright in each hand, palms facing each other, and rest the tips of the weights on the thighs.

  2. Use your legs to rock back so that you're lying flat on the bench. Move the weights up to your chest. Now bring your palms parallel (the backs of the hands are facing you), weights at the level of your bust, shoulder width apart. Take a deep breath.

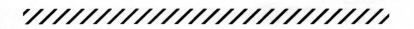

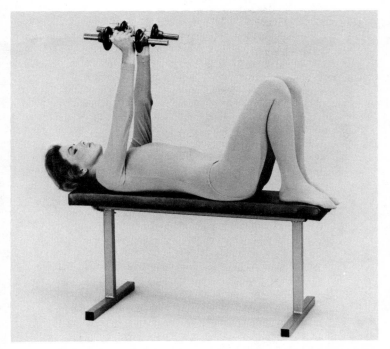

3. *Blow out your breath and push the weights straight up, with your elbows locked and your arms extended directly above you at mid-chest level, not over your shoulders, not over your stomach. Breathe in as you lower the weights with control, bringing your elbows down toward the floor for a full extension.*

Weight: 5–7½ lbs. each dumbbell: dumbbell bars alone or with two 1¼-lb. plates on each.

Reps: 3 sets of 10.

Note: *After completing the reps, drop the weights to the floor before sitting up; do not bring them up with you.*

TWO

CLOSE GRIP DUMBBELL PRESS///////

for the pectorals

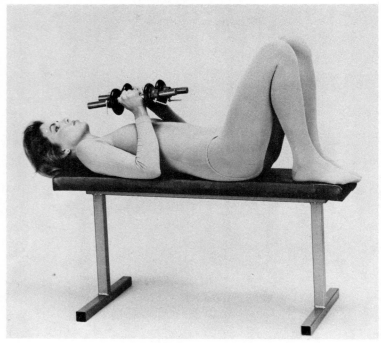

1. Using the same starting position as before, lie back with palms facing each other, dumbbells touching lengthwise. Take a deep breath.

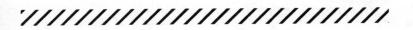

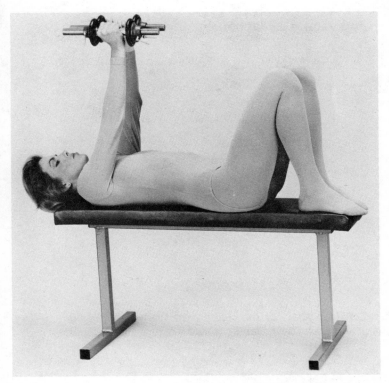

2. Blow out and push the weights straight up, directly over mid-chest, keeping the weights pressed together as you raise them. Breathe in as you lower the weights to mid-chest.

Weight: 5–7½ lbs. each dumbbell: dumbbell bars alone or with two 1¼-lb. plates on each.

Reps: 3 sets of 10.

Note: *Again, release the weights to the floor before sitting up; do not bring them up with you.*

THREE
DUMBBELL FLIES'/////////////////

for the pectorals

Variation #1: Flat bench.

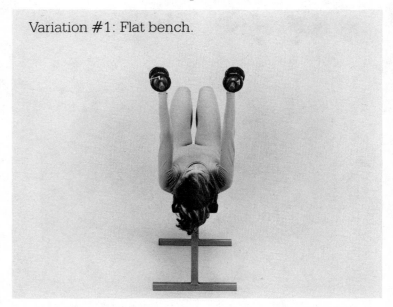

1. *Lying back on the bench, raise the weights straight up over your shoulders, palms facing in, arms straight, and elbows locked.*

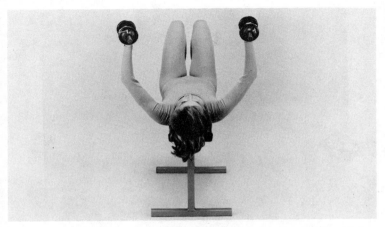

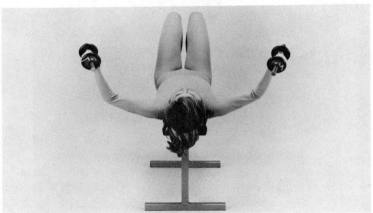

2. *Inhale and bring the weights out to the sides in a semicircle until they are just below shoulder level. Bend your elbows to ease the tension and get the widest extension possible.*

3. *Exhale and bring your arms back to the starting position, elbows locked.*

////////////////////////////////////.

Variation #2: Inclined bench.

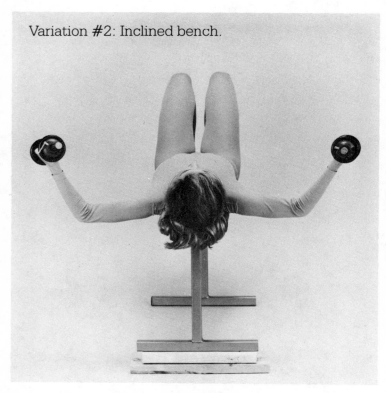

Place a two-by-four board under the top end of the bench to elevate it slightly. Repeat the flies. The change in position works the upper pectorals.

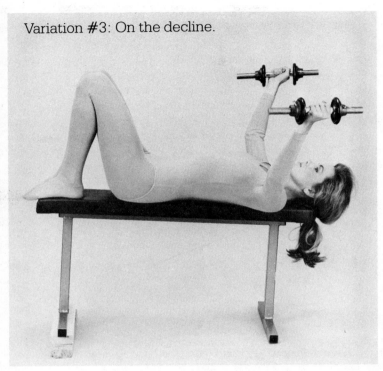

Variation #3: On the decline.

Place the two-by-four at the other end of the bench and repeat the flies. The change in position works the lower pectorals.

DO ALL THREE VARIATIONS OF THE EXERCISE!

Weight: 5–7½ lbs. each dumbbell: dumbbell bars alone or with two 1¼-lb. plates on each.

Reps: 2 sets of 10 for each variation.

Note: *After each set, lower the weights to the floor before sitting up.*

FOUR

THE PULLOVER /////////////////////

for the pectorals, the serratus, and especially the deltoids

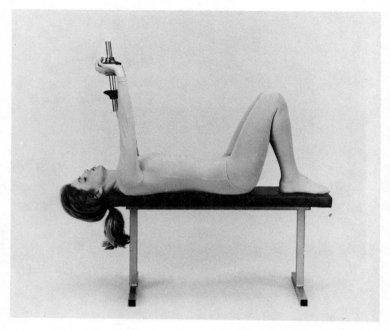

1. Lie back on the bench with your head slightly off the end of the bench to get a full extension during the exercise. Grip the top of one dumbbell with the crook of your right hand and place your left hand over the right. Raise your arms and hold the weight just over your head.

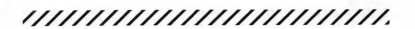

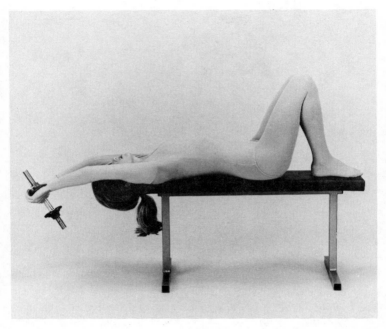

2. Take a deep breath and extend your arms behind your head and back toward the floor. You should feel your back lift off the bench slightly. Exhale as you bring your arms back to the starting position.

Weight: one 10-lb. dumbbell: a dumbbell bar with two plates, each 2¹/₂ lbs.

Reps: 2 sets of 10.

Note: After the reps, drop the weight to the floor before sitting up; do not bring it up with you.

FIVE

BENT KNEE ROWS///////////////////,

for the latissimus dorsi muscles of the back

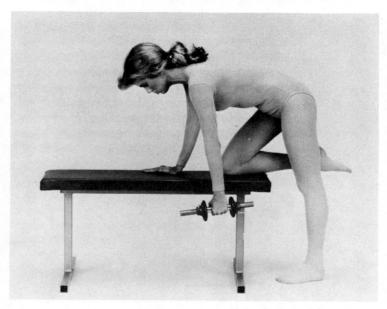

1. *Stand facing the foot of your bench and place your right knee on it securely for support. Your left leg stays on the ground. Bend over, placing your right hand high enough on the bench to extend your back into a flat, tabletop position. Pick up the dumbbell with your left hand and hold it, arm straight. Take a deep breath.*

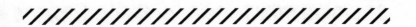

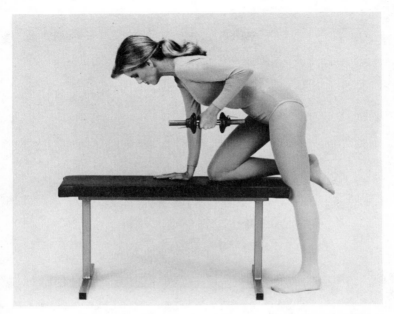

2. Bring the weight up toward the left side of your rib cage by bending the arm, elbow close to your body, not out to the side. (Keep your wrist relaxed; use the arm, not the wrist, to lift the weight.) Lower the arm. Exhale as you raise the weight, inhale as you lower it. You should feel the pull along the length of your side. Do all the reps and then repeat the exercise on the right side, left knee and hand on the bench.

Weight: one 10-lb. dumbbell (a dumbbell bar with two plates, each 2¹/₂ lbs.)

Reps: 3 sets of 10 on each side.

Note: *Before switching sides and after completing the reps, drop the weight to the floor; do not carry it with you as you change positions.*

SIX

STANDING ROWS/////////////////.

for the latissimus dorsi

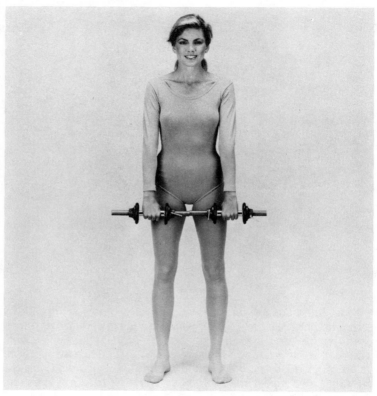

1. *Standing straight, shoulders back, feet slightly apart, hold a dumbbell in each hand, palms facing the front of the thighs. Dumbbells touch end to end. Take a deep breath.*

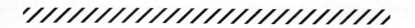

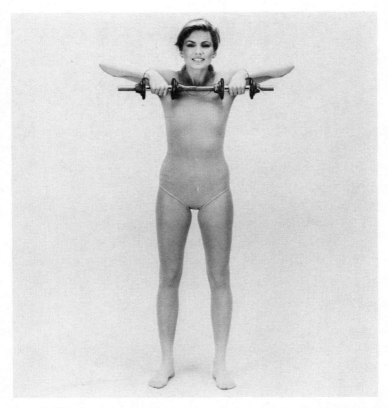

2. Exhale and raise the weights straight up to your chin. (Keep the weights together.) Bend your elbows out to the sides and up. Inhale as you lower the weights. You should definitely feel the pull of the muscles in your upper back.

Weight: 5–7½ lbs. each dumbbell: dumbbell bars only or with two 1¼-lb. plates on each.

Reps: 2 sets of 10.

SEVEN

LATERAL RAISES///////////////////

*for the deltoid muscles in the shoulders and
the trapezius*

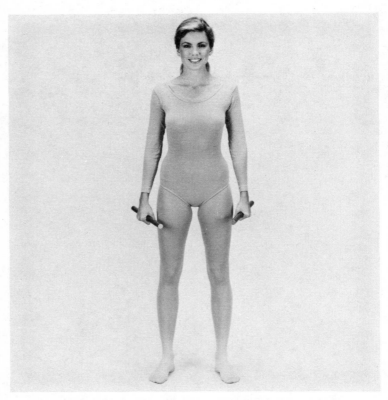

1. *Stand with your feet slightly apart, shoulders back, arms
straight at your sides and relaxed. Hold a dumbbell (bar only) in
each hand with palms facing in. Take a deep breath.*

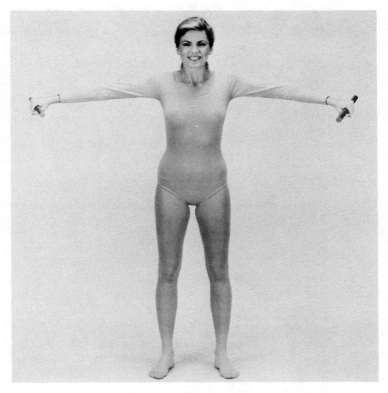

2. *Raise your arms straight out to the sides until they are parallel to the floor at the level of your shoulders. Exhale as you raise the arms, breathe in as you lower them. Be sure to keep your shoulders squared and still.*

Weight: 5 lbs. each dumbbell: dumbbell bars only.

Reps: 2 sets of 10.

EIGHT

ALTERNATE FRONT RAISES///////////.

for the front of the deltoids

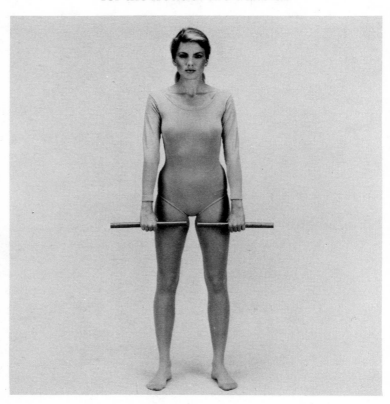

1. Stand in the same starting position as in exercise seven. Bring the arms forward so that the palms face the front of the thighs. Relax your arms to extend them fully; don't tighten up in the wrists. Take a deep breath.

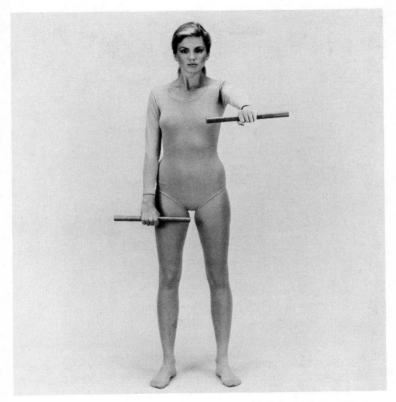

2. Exhale and raise your right arm straight out in front of you to shoulder level. Inhale as you lower the right arm, then exhale, and raise the left arm. Continue to alternate arms until you have completed all the reps.

Weight: 5 lbs. each dumbbell: dumbbell bars only.

Reps: 2 sets of 10 for a total of 10 raises of each arm.

NINE

FLAT-BACK RAISES ////////////////////

for the rear of the deltoids

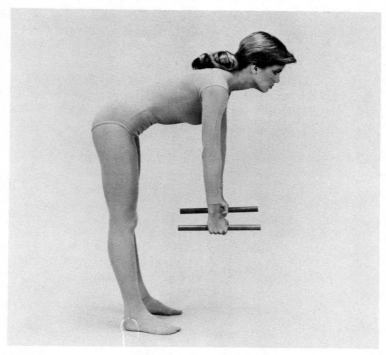

1. Stand with your feet apart and bend from the waist to make a flat, tabletop position with your back. Hold a dumbbell in each hand, arms straight to the floor. Take a deep breath.

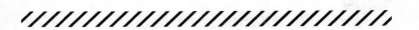

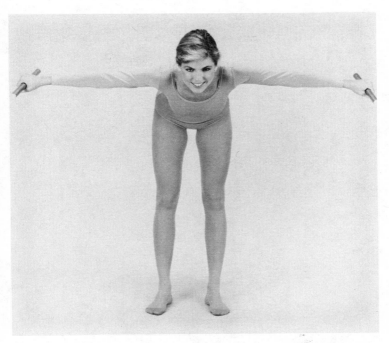

2. *Exhale and raise the weights out to the sides, making one long line straight with your shoulders. (Only the arms move.) Do not lift up your back. Inhale as you lower your arms to the starting position.*

Weight: 5 lbs. each dumbbell: dumbbell bars only.

Reps: 2 sets of 10.

TEN

ALTERNATE DUMBBELL CURLS///////.

for the biceps

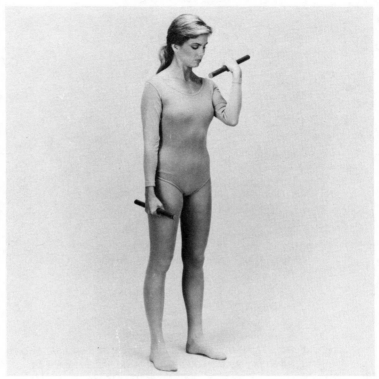

1. Stand with your feet slightly apart, shoulders back, back straight. Hold a dumbbell in each hand, palms against the thighs. Take a deep breath. Exhale and bring your right palm toward your face and curl it up to your right shoulder.

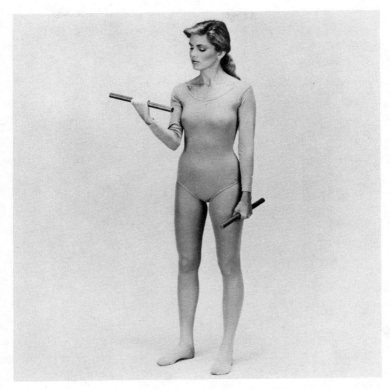

2. Inhale as you lower the right arm and exhale as you raise the left one. Continue to alternate arms until you have completed all the reps.

Concentrate on keeping your shoulders square; don't lean into the weight to make the exercise easier. Stay steady; don't swing or jerk your arms.

Weight: 5 lbs. each dumbbell: dumbbell bars only.

Reps: 2 sets of 10 for a total of 10 curls on each side.

ELEVEN

SUPPORTED DUMBBELL CURLS//////////

for the biceps

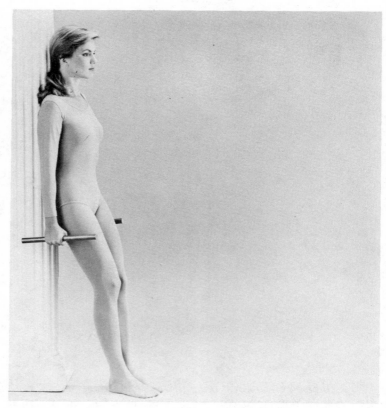

1. Stand against an open door frame or along the corner of two walls for support. Your back and head should touch the support, and your legs should be slightly in front. Keep your back straight at all times. Take a deep breath.

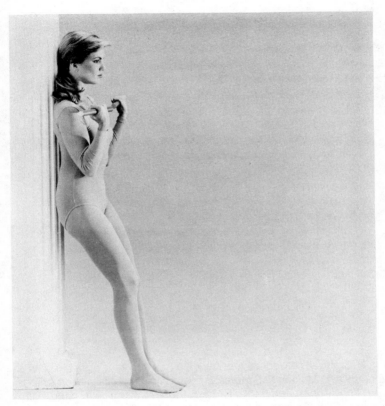

2. Curl both arms simultaneously as you exhale. Feel your biceps flexing as the weights touch your shoulders. Inhale as you lower your arms.

Weight: 5 lbs. each dumbbell: dumbbell bars only.

Reps: 2 sets of 10 curls.

TWELVE

FLAT-BACK TRICEP EXTENSION//////////

for the triceps

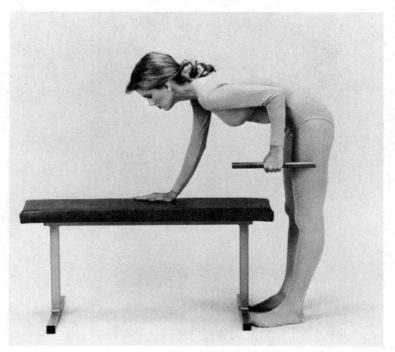

1. Stand at the foot of your bench and place your right hand on it for support. Make a flat, tabletop position with your back. Your legs are slightly apart and bent. Hold a dumbbell in your left hand, palm forward. The upper arm is along your left side with your elbow bent at your waist. (The forearm makes a right angle with the upper arm.) Take a deep breath.

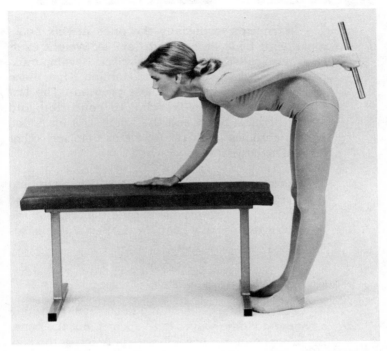

2. Exhale and straighten your forearm behind you to push up the weight. The forearm is the only part of your body that moves. You should feel the action in the back of your upper arm.

3. Inhale and bring the forearm back to the starting position, elbow locked throughout. Do both sets on the left arm, then reverse your position to work the right.

Weight: one 5-lb. dumbbell bar.

Reps: 2 sets of 10 on each side.

WORKING OUT WITH AEROBICS

Warm-ups, especially the ones in this book, make your body limber and flexible. Weight exercises, also called resistance exercises, develop muscles and increase strength and stamina. They make up two-thirds of a total fitness program. The last element is aerobic exercise to condition and strengthen the heart and the lungs. (As an added bonus, aerobics work off fat faster than any other form of activity.)

Aerobic sports include running, biking, jumping rope, cross-country skiing, fast dancing, rowing, and swimming. All are excellent conditioners, but the last two are especially good for the pectoral muscles and deserve a closer look.

Swimming

For most of us, swimming means lolling around a pool or dodging waves in the ocean, but the benefits of swimming only come with laps across the pool or strokes swum parallel to the shore. In the beginning, your body may tire easily when you log those laps, but with practice you will be able to build up to 20, and then 30 minutes of swimming two or three times a week.

Water cushions your body, so injuries are rare. For this reason, swimming is the preferred sport.

The following tips will make swimming a pleasure:

- Wear a tank suit for comfort; a strapless *maillot* will be swimming around your waist with your second stroke.

- Wear goggles to protect your eyes when swimming in a chlorinated pool; noseplugs, if you wish.

- Always wash your hair after swimming to remove a pool's chlorine or the ocean's salt, even if you wear a cap.

- Swim three times a week for best results.

Rowing

As a team sport, you can't beat rowing for fun and fitness. But few of us have access to a rowing team! Rowing machines for the home have made this sport more accessible on an individual basis. The compact home models, costing less than a year's membership at a health club, are excellent for aerobic training. Look for models that work your legs and arms simultaneously. Be sure to follow the manufacturer's instructions. Wear a sports bra and support sneakers for each workout.

Note: Before any aerobic exercise, be sure to warm up your muscles; afterward, stretching exercises to cool you down are a must.

ADDED ADVICE FOR FITNESS

Though you are concentrating on your upper torso, it is important not to neglect the rest of your body. Be sure to start an aerobic program for all-over fitness: they all exercise the muscles in the legs and buttocks. To complete your weight training, consider adding other weight exercises that work the abductors and adductors in the thighs and the gluteal muscles in your bottom. Remember that any individual muscle group can be developed with the proper exercise.

3. DRESSING RIGHT

Much of a woman's anguish over her breasts comes from her sense about whether her figure meets the requirements of current fashion. In fact, most of us are so influenced by fashion trends that each season creates new anxiety: "Are my legs ready for a change in hem length?" "Is my waist small enough for the cinched look?"

It's time to turn the tables on those who dictate fashion. Starting today, you decide the styles you will wear to flatter your figure, and don't let yourself be swayed. (You can be sure that most men won't care or even know if you're in fashion—a man admires a woman who looks like she belongs in her clothes.) Part of developing your individuality is selecting clothes that do you justice, rather than playing the part of a mannequin for someone's whimsical designs.

Your bust can be improved with the right clothing styles as successfully as other parts of your body. Here are the guidelines you need to know.

FASHIONS TO FLATTER A SMALL BOSOM

Generally, avoid thin, clingy fabrics that emphasize small proportions. Chose crisp fabrics such as cotton and linen, in heavier textures. Layer a shirt, sweater, and jacket for more dimension.

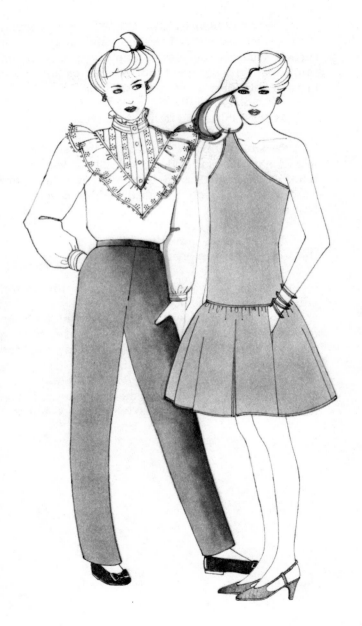

Shirts and blouses. Select tops with interesting details such as pleated tuxedo shirts and lacy or ruffled Victorian blouses. Camp shirts in popular, bright patterns are good. Puffed sleeves and exaggerated shoulders add dimension, too.

Avoid T-shirts and tightly fitted turtlenecks.

Sweaters. Textured sweaters in fluffy wools, like mohair, *blouson* styles (especially if you have a thick waist), and fisherman cable-stitch knits are good choices. Sweaters with three-dimensional details are great, too.

Avoid boyish, crew-neck Shetland sweaters—they give an ironing board look!

Dresses. Smocked dresses with interesting stitching over the bodice, dresses with exaggerated shoulders, or bare-shoulder, camisole, or tank-top dresses are the most flattering. Dresses with a dropped waistline are great, because they steal the eye away from the bosom.

Swimwear. A strapless *maillot* is best. If you have a thick waist, choose one with *blouson* styling.

FASHIONS TO FLATTER A LARGE BOSOM

Generally, start with a bra that has a natural shape and excellent underwire construction. The best place to shop for foundations is at a specialty store, rather than in a large department store. Get to know your *corsetière* and take advantage of her experience. Don't be embarrassed to let her help you—that's her business. A perfect-fitting bra will hide unattractive bulges. You can find beautiful styles and colors available now in all sizes.

Shirts and blouses. The ease of a soft pullover is more flattering than a stiff shirt, as long as you choose fabrics with definition (two-ply knits rather than single-ply). When you do want a blouse, choose soft fabrics such as silk; a fine, thin wool; and pliable cotton blends. Necklines are important; choose U or V shapes, square or scoop necks. Never wear crew or round necklines or collarless shirts. Avoid fussy details; stick with classic styling. Deep, rich colors work better than pastels or prints.

Sweaters and jackets. Soft cowl-neck and shawl-collar sweaters in thinner wools and acrylics are best; never wear a turtleneck. Sweater jackets and cardigans are more attractive than blazers, especially if you wear a wrap sweater in place of a shirt and blazer. A *blouson* sweater is fine as long as the knit is not too bulky.

When you want to wear a jacket or blazer, choose an unconstructed style that doesn't have to be buttoned. Chanel-style squared-off jackets work, too. Pulling the fabric on a jacket across the bust to close it emphasizes a large measurement; wearing an open jacket minimizes it.

Dresses. Avoid smock dresses that will fall from the bust like a huge tent; wear a belt to define your waistline for contrast. Choose dresses with the same attention to neckline you show to buying blouses and tops. A wrapdress is a good choice. A shirtdress worn belted is another. (If your waistline is on the thick side, you can still wear a belt, simply choose the narrowest ones you can find in colors and fabrics that best match your clothes.)

Rich colors are better than light pastels and prints. Soft knits that move with you are better than stiff, heavy fabrics.

Swimwear. Halter suits that offer support without preformed cups are a good choice; those cut low in the back are more attractive than even the skimpiest bikini.

Strapless clothes. Large-chested women have difficulty wearing strapless clothes (bandeau tops, one-shoulder dresses, camisoles, etc.). The answer is a lingerie garment called a *bustier* or corselette. With more support than the average strapless bra (which often makes its way to your waist in an hour!), the *bustier* is effective and beautiful, especially when made of Poirette lace. It fastens from bosom to waist, creating perfect definition under all clothes.

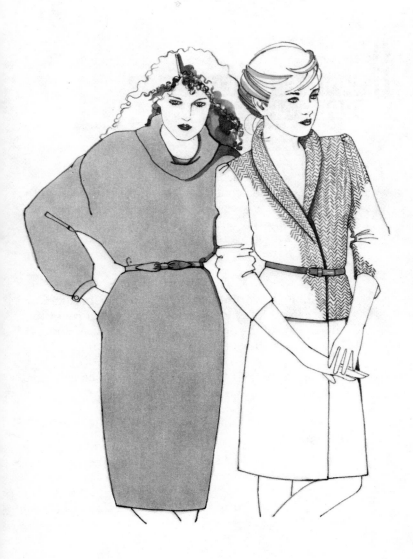

HOW TO FLATTER HEAVY UPPER ARMS

Follow these guidelines when selecting your clothes:

1. Choose blouses, sweaters, and dresses with raglan, batwing, or dolman sleeves, which camouflage and flatter. Choose full-length or three-quarter sleeves; avoid sleeveless tank tops, shell tops, camisoles, spaghetti straps, and sleeves that bind at your middle arm.

2. For evening glamour, choose blouses or dresses with off-the-shoulder sleeves that cover the fullest part of the upper arm. Wear strapless clothing and drape a shawl across your shoulders.

3. Avoid very thin, clingy fabrics such as nylon and jersey; they outline every bulge.

4. Use fashion to look your best. Never let it use you!

4. BEAUTIFUL BREASTS

Beauty and beauty care don't stop at your neckline. The rest of your body deserves the same kind of attention you give your face.

HOW TO PAMPER YOUR SKIN

Caring for your breasts doesn't call for special (or expensive) products, just a little attention. Breast creams, like those designed just for the neck or just for the forehead or just for the left side of your nose, aren't necessary. A good, light moisturizer is fine.

Cleansing. When bathing or showering, gently sponge the skin of your breasts with a soft mitt or cloth; save your loofah for elbows and rough patches on the upper arms. Be sure to clean under the folds of the breasts, especially after exercise, to remove perspiration.

Moisturizing. While your skin is still wet, smooth on your lotion or moisturizer. Let your body dry naturally, then buff with a towel. Be sure to absorb any moisture. If you wish, finish with baby powder or scented talc.

A bit of cocoa butter or lanolin on the areolae is recommended for women who are pregnant or nursing or whose skin tends to be quite dry.

$\mathbb{S}$OLVING BEAUTY PROBLEMS

Stretch marks. From the day we are born, gravity starts working against us. As we grow older, the weight of the breasts stretches the skin, causing these slight marks.

Wearing a good bra that supports the breasts helps postpone stretch marks, but little can be done about getting rid of existing ones. This is the kind of flaw only *you* notice and should therefore be put out of your mind.

Unwanted beauty marks. Though these, too, are a beauty woe women worry about unnecessarily, a plastic surgeon should be consulted about any marks you would like removed. More important, you should notify your doctor immediately if you notice any change in a mole or any bleeding from it.

Unwanted hair. Often one or a few hairs can be found on the breasts, especially around the areolae. These can be removed with tweezers or a *careful* whisk with a ladies' razor. Persistent growth can be permanently removed by a certified, well-recommended electrologist. (Any hair growing from a mole or beauty mark should be snipped off with scissors, not plucked or shaved.)

Breakouts. These can occur on your chest and back, even after adolescence. Wash with an antibacterial soap only, nothing perfumed or containing oil. Avoid synthetic fabrics that don't *breathe* and that can irritate an already bothersome condition. Visit a dermatologist if the problem persists.

Dermatitis. This irritation, which most often strikes in the form of dishwater hands, can cause reddish blotches around your bra line. Often the cause is perspiration and its ensuing bacteria. Always be sure to wear a cotton sports bra when exercising, to wash it after every workout and to shower afterward. Seeking professional help is the best remedy for a persistent problem and well worth the effort and the cost.

Sunburn. First-time topless sunbathers are often unpleasantly surprised at how easily the skin of the breasts can burn. Thinner skinned than the other parts of your body, the breasts are rarely exposed to the sun and have no resistance to the sun's strong rays. If you are planning an exotic vacation in the sun, take the same precautions that you would—or *should* —with the rest of your body: use a very effective sunscreen.

A strong sun can burn through even the fabric of a swimsuit, especially a black one. Apply your sunscreen all over before putting on your suit. (Check the product label to be sure it is nonstaining.)

YOUR BEAUTY QUESTIONS ANSWERED

Q. *Does weight gain or loss affect the size of the breasts?*

A. Yes, because the breasts are made up of fatty tissue. When you gain weight, the areas of your body with a predisposition to fat (thighs, buttocks, hips, upper arms, and breasts) will show the added pounds. When you lose weight, the body uses up fat stores drawn from all these areas as well.

But because the size of your bust is in part determined by heredity, the changes can't be controlled precisely. Don't let concern over your bust measurement keep you from achieving and maintaining your ideal weight. That's when you're the healthiest.

Q. *Can pregnancy and/or nursing harm my breasts?*

A. No. We forget that the pure function of our breasts is to nurse our babies. It is distressing to hear women say they will deny their infants breast feeding because it may ruin their bustline. Nursing actually helps restore the figure they were so afraid of losing! The only special care required is wearing a well constructed bra and giving a bit of extra attention to cleansing. The bond that nursing creates between mother and child is unmatched by any other relationship.

Q. *Should I give myself a breast exam every month?*

A. Yes. Because you probably have a medical checkup only once every year or two, it's important to be aware of your body between visits to the doctor. A breast exam is easy, quick, and painless.

At your next office visit, ask your doctor to show you how it is done, then do it at home, once a month, after each menstrual cycle. (If you don't want to wait, your local branch of the American Cancer Society can provide you with a pamphlet that gives this information.)

5. INSTANT IMPROVEMENT

In the past few decades, the science of plastic surgery has become an art. It is possible to redesign any part of the body along shapelier lines. More perfect breasts are available not just to Hollywood actresses but to any woman who can afford the operation. But it is just that, an operation complete with hospital stay, hospital bills, a visit to the operating room, and all the discomfort that that entails. Having breast surgery calls for very careful thought.

Why consider surgery at all? Surgery is, to date, the only sure way to radically change your bustline. This is especially important for women with very large breasts who suffer from backaches and other painful symptoms. Breast reduction surgery can reshape contours for your physical and aesthetic well-being.

Opting for surgery to *increase* the size of your breasts is more complex. You must be satisfied with your reasons, even if that means seeking professional advice. Be sure that you aren't judging yourself strictly in terms of your physical appearance. Having bigger breasts might make you more attractive but shouldn't be crucial to your feelings of self-worth. Ask yourself what you hope the surgery will accomplish for you, then realistically evaluate your answers.

FACTS ABOUT SURGICAL TECHNIQUES

Breast enlargement. In this operation, an implant filled with silicone solution is inserted beneath your natural tissues. The size of the implant used will be determined by you and your surgeon in proportion to your figure. The incision can be made along the lower outline of the areolae or under the fold of each breast, depending on your build. The operation, which can be performed under general anesthesia, takes about three hours. You will be hospitalized for only a few days.

Healing time is approximately two weeks, though a temporary loss of sensitivity can last longer. Your doctor will clue you in to other side effects to expect during your recovery period. The stitches will leave thin scars that do fade in time.

Breast reduction. In this operation, fatty tissue and excess skin are removed from the breasts to reshape them. Depending on the amount of reduction, the areolae may have to be repositioned, making the operation and the healing period somewhat longer than for breast enlargement. The incisions will likely be made around the natural outline of the areolae; this calls for a number of stitches, but, again, the scars fade in time.

Your surgeon will show you many before-and-after photographs to help you understand the procedure and the intended results. Be sure he discusses all the possible side effects of the operation. These can include the inability to breast feed.

Though this is a corrective surgical technique that will eliminate the often underestimated problem of pendulous breasts, it is still major surgery and should be considered very carefully.

CHOOSING A PLASTIC SURGEON

Once you have made the decision to pursue the possibility of cosmetic surgery, your next step is selecting a surgeon. In the hands of a gifted doctor, truly dramatic results are possible. Because this field of specialization is lucrative, there is no shortage of available surgeons. That is why you, as the consumer, must be extremely discerning.

A surgeon's reputation is often based on recommendations. Ask only doctors you trust for assistance in finding a surgeon. Don't limit yourself to one surgeon. Investigate two or three. Make an appointment for a consultation with each of those you're considering. Listen to what each doctor has to say and then ask questions. Evaluate their answers just as you evaluated your own reasons for electing the surgery. It is very easy to be intimidated by a doctor, especially a surgeon, but you must remember that the ultimate decision is yours.

Once you are satisfied with the surgeon you have interviewed, consider once more the decision you have made. If the surgeon had any reservations about your operation, think over your reasoning once again. Review the surgical procedure, the facts about the healing, and any possible complications. Use all the information before you to make an educated, well-thought-out decision you can live with happily.

/ / / / / / / / / /

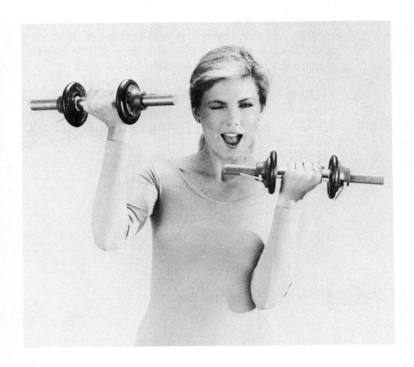

ABOUT THE AUTHORS

Julie Davis is the author of twenty-six books, the first of which she wrote at age sixteen. Her nonfiction titles include five celebrity how-to's co-authored with singer Marie Osmond, model Beverly Johnson, actress Arlene Dahl, and two noted skin-care experts, Janet Sartin and Irma Shorell.

Regina Larkin's keen interest in body awareness and fitness has led her to dual careers in dance performance and physical health. She has danced with a number of professional companies and is currently a member of the Joyce Trisler Danscompany in New York. Regina is on the dance faculty of Adelphi University and also teaches at the Joyce Trisler Danscompany School. She has toured extensively, performing and giving demonstrations and teaching techniques of body toning and alignment in such places as the Kennedy Center in Washington, D.C., the Georges Pompidou Centre in Paris, and at numerous colleges and universities.